Gum Disease:

Care & Treatment

Gum Disease:

Care & Treatment

Completely Revised – 2015 Edition

Howard B. Marshall, D.D.S

Revised 2015 Edition:
ISBN 13: 978-1508792567   ISBN 10: 1508792569

This publication is designed to provide accurate and authoritative information in regard to the subject matter covered. It is sold with the understanding that
neither the author(s) nor the publisher is engaged in rendering dental, or other professional service.
If dental advice or other expert assistance is required,
the services of a competent professional should be sought.

PRINTED IN THE UNITED STATES OF AMERICA

AUTHOR AND PUBLISHER'S NOTE

Every effort has been made to ensure that the information contained in this book is complete and accurate. This 2015 edition updates the 2011 edition. However, neither the author nor the publisher is engaged in rendering professional advice or services to the individual reader. The ideas, procedures, and suggestions contained in this book are not intended as a substitute for consulting with your dentist or dental specialist. All matters regarding your dental health require dental supervision. Neither the author nor the publisher shall be liable or responsible for any loss, injury, or damage allegedly arising from any information or suggestion in this book.

DEDICATION

This book is dedicated, first and foremost, to my mentors: Dr. D. Walter Cohen, Dean Emeritus, University of Pennsylvania, School of Dental Medicine, Medical College of Pennsylvania, President Emeritus, Medical College of Pennsylvania, Chancellor Emeritus, Diplomat of the American Board of Periodontology, and its Chairman in 1971-1972, Editor Emeritus of Compendium of Continuing Education in General Dentistry; and Dr. Henry M. Goldman, deceased, Founder and Dean Emeritus of the Henry M. Goldman School of Dental Medicine, Boston University.

Secondly, I dedicate this book to the memory of my parents, Leon and Florine Marshall, for their sacrifices, without which I could not have become a periodontist.

Lastly, I dedicate this book to my dental colleagues for their ongoing efforts to improve our profession to better serve mankind, and to my patients, whose many questions inspired me to write the original book and this completely updated version.

ABOUT THE AUTHOR

Dr. Marshall has been in practice for over thirty years. He originally graduated from the University of Pennsylvania School of Dental Medicine, followed by a second year of training at Boston University's Graduate School of Medicine, Department of Stomatology. He then entered the United States Air Force, and served for two years as a captain in the dental services department.

Upon return to the United States, Dr. Marshall limited his practice exclusively to Periodontics for 16 years. Subsequently, because of his additional background as a highly trained sculptor and painter, he elected to become expert in cosmetic and restorative dentistry. Today, in addition to his periodontal background, he has over twenty years of experience in restorative and cosmetic dentistry. He has taken well over one hundred postgraduate courses. He has placed over 6000 dental implants. Where necessary, he has rebuilt the bone into which the needed implants were placed. He has also restored the teeth by placing crowns on top of the implants. He practices 3 days/week. See his website.

He is Chairman and CEO or Oro-Health International, Inc., a company whose first product is a one visit, one hour tooth replacement system, requiring no surgery, and is probably going to only cost the patient 50% of other treatment approaches. The product will be ready sometime in 2016 for the dental profession. Oro-Health International, Inc. is also working on some other very innovative products. They should be ready about 2017.

Dr. Marshall has not only rebuilt many mouths, but also created beautiful smiles. He has worked in cooperation with other expert dental teams of specialists, or as the periodontal or implant surgeon in conjunction with a restorative dental specialist. He believes very strongly that patients should get total comprehensive treatment planning, and that, where health and budget allow, dentists and patients are best served by state of the art techniques. He also believes in preventing future disease, and in counseling with advanced nutritional information for a patient's overall health.

Dr. Marshall's 2 previous dental books for the public were: (1980) "How to Save Your Teeth-The Preventive Approach.", (2009) "Dental Health & Treatment – Dental Cosmetics & Beauty", and 2011, Gum Disease: Care & Treatment.

He has been awarded over 10 patents for his research on the one-visit tooth replacement system, which he hopes to introduce to the marketplace sometime in the next two years.

Dr. Marshall practices in New York City, New York, USA.

TABLE OF CONTENTS

Author and publisher's note

Dedication

About the author

1. Where Bad Breath and Gum Disease Come from

2. Frequently Asked Questions about Bleeding Gums

3. Treatment of Bad Breath and Early Gum Disease

4. The Many Causes of Bad Breath

5. How Decay and Gum Disease Progress in the Adult

6. A Good Dental Examination Includes The Following

7. How to Get the Proper Treatment Plan for Your Mouth

8. Advantages of Early Periodontal Treatment

9. Everything You Need To Know about Different Treatment Approaches

10. The Dental Specialties

11. Implants

12. Most Frequent Questions about Implants

13. Frequently Asked General Dental Questions

Conclusion

References

CHAPTER ONE

BAD BREATH AND BLEEDING GUMS

Introduction:

How Many People Have Periodontal Disease (Gum Disease)?

Gum disease (and really, disease in the bone supporting the teeth) is nearly a universal problem. It is found in every country. Early signs of periodontal disease are frequently evident in the twenties. Advanced destruction is commonly observed after the age of 40 years. In countries like China, and India, over 90% of adults have some disease.

As people get older, one often finds gum recession. In the US, a 6 year survey finished in 1994, showed 35% of participants had gum inflammation and bone loss based on pocket depth. Later studies showed over 50% loss. An even greater number (64%) were experiencing the disease when it was based on loss of attachment of the gum to the root.

So we can see that a considerable number of people in the United States are suffering from periodontal disease and are not aware of it. It does not produce pain, but can lead to extensive bone loss and, later, loss of teeth if not treated. Considering the past 50 years of available data, there has fortunately been a reduction in the total number of people in the US who would be classified as having periodontal disease, especially of the severe form. This does not hold true for immigrants from foreign countries that did not have the opportunity to get dental care before moving to the US. Very often these newer US residents have much more severe periodontal breakdown and loss of teeth.

Recognizing Gum Disease: How can you recognize gingivitis (gum) or periodontal disease (disease of tooth-supporting bone)? Why might you need periodontal treatment?

Here are the signs to help you recognize your own gum disease

1. Bleeding gums
2. Puffy gums
3. Shiny or swollen gums
4. Bad breath
5. Pink toothbrush
6. Enlarged gums with a reddish color
7. Gum recession
8. Spaces between the teeth where no spaces previously existed
9. Loose teeth
10. Shifting teeth
11. Gum abscesses—puffy, enlarged soreness of the gum
12. Itchiness of the gum
13. Tenderness of the gum

CONTOUR OF NORMAL, RECEDED, AND INFLAMED GUM

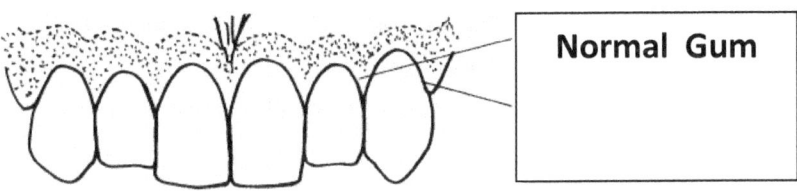

Normal Gum

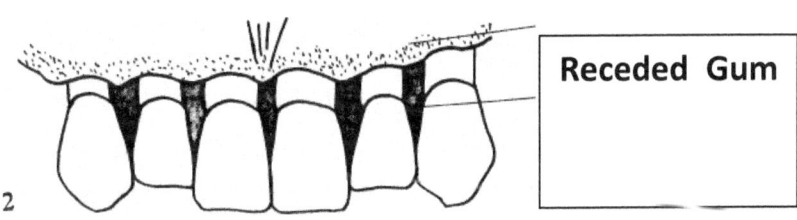

Receded Gum

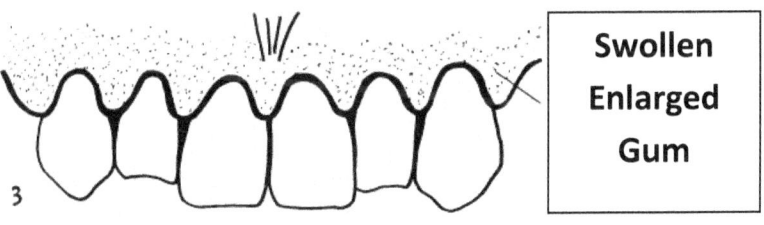

Swollen Enlarged Gum

Disease of the Teeth, Gum, and Bone

Gum disease starts with breakdown of the gum and bone caused by bacteria living in the gum space next to the tooth. This dense bacterial jungle is called **biofilm**. Your tooth sits in a hole in your jawbone called a socket, separated from the socket wall by a thin membrane or **ligament**. This periodontal ligament seems to act as a sling and hydraulic system. It prevents the tooth when you bite from being overly squeezed into the socket. Healthy gum is attached to the tooth just above the bone, like a banana peel over a banana.

There is a space between the gum lining and tooth called a sulcus. It is very tiny, about 1-2 mm deep (1/8 inch). At the bottom of this space, there is a tight adaptation of the gum lining to the tooth enamel (the white part of your tooth). The tight adaptation is called the epithelial attachment. Just under this, there are millions of fibers attaching the gum tissue to the root. See the drawing on the next page.

The gum space is critically important because it fills up with bacteria very soon after the tooth erupts. These bacteria, if not removed by brushing and flossing, irritate the cells lining the gum. This causes the lining cells to swell and separate. Although your gum space always has some bacteria, as they increase in number and type, they cause your gum lining to breakdown and bleed, like an ulcer. When the lining of the gum space becomes diseased and bleeds, the gum space often deepens and is called a **pocket**.

As the gum lining continues to break down, the fibers just below the **epithelial attachment** also break down. These fibers are just above the bone and form part of the gum so once they have broken down the bone itself begins to dissolve.

Some Important Facts about Bacterial Plaque and Biofilm

There are hundreds of different kinds of bacteria in the mouth. Some cause periodontal disease and some cause decay. Only a few kinds are considered most responsible for causing tooth decay. Certain bacteria have the ability to break down sugars into acids. Some bacteria also produce a complicated sticky material which allows bacteria to hold tightly to your tooth surface. Other bacteria stick right to the tooth surface itself and work directly on decaying enamel. Still others settle on the backs of the earlier bacterial arrivals. Thus bacteria live in a mesh of many layers called **biofilm**.

Gingivitis, which is an inflammation of the gum but has not yet caused bone loss, is reversible. Periodontal disease is not reversible. The pathogenic bacteria that cause periodontal disease live deep in the diseased gum space (pocket) and generally do best in an environment that has very little oxygen.

How do these bacteria do their damage? They produce enzymes that dissolve protein, produce nutrients for other bacteria, and destroy the gum lining, connective tissue, and bone. They lie in a slimy meshwork composed of saliva, dextran (the sticky material), other bacteria, food, and salivary breakdown products. Plaque is much thicker than saliva. **Plaque (pronounced plak) and biofilm are the most important words to remember in this book.**

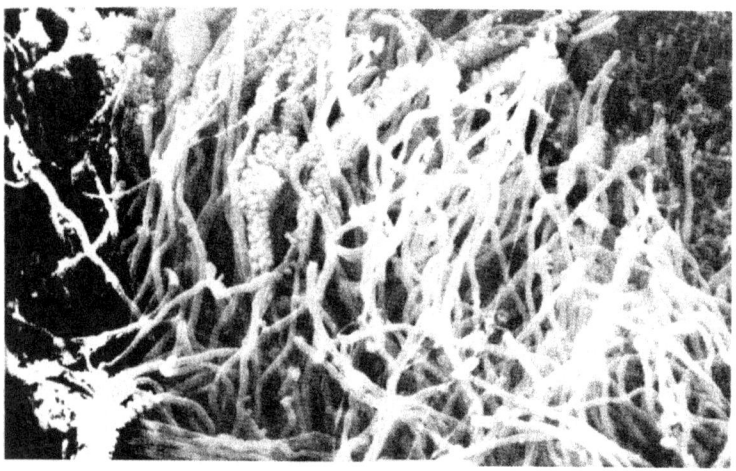

PLAQUE SHOWING BACTERIAL FORMS UNDER HIGH MAGNIFICATION

The Gum Disease Process Can Lead to Severe Medical Conditions. How?

Let's first examine Gingivitis – Inflammation of the Gum

We said earlier that the diseased gum space (pocket) occurs when your gum lining and the connective tissue fibers under the gum lining breakdown, forming a periodontal pocket.

When this pocket develops, tooth brushing or eating hard foods might cause your gums to bleed. **This bleeding is not normal**. When the bacteria are in the early phase of destroying the gum lining and the connective tissue, we call this stage gingivitis. In your mouth, you can see this stage if your tissue is red, shiny, flabby, or tender, looks slightly puffy or swollen between the teeth, and, frequently, bleeds easily. This stage is produced by bacterial plaque (biofilm) and is reversible with proper treatment.

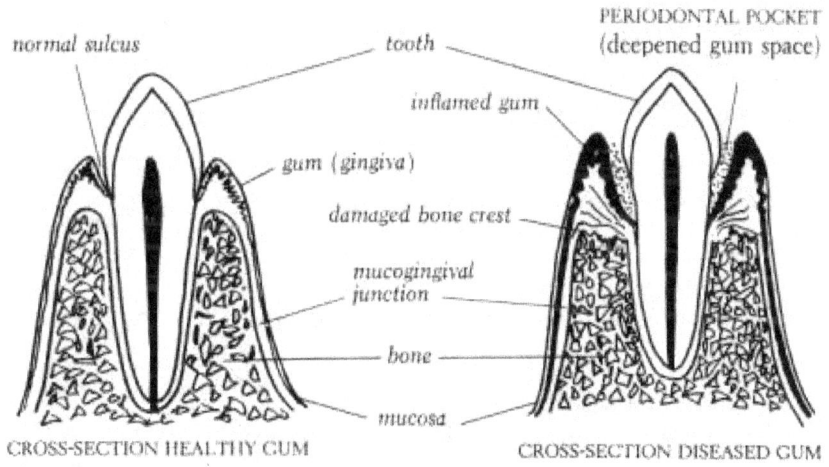

CROSS-SECTION HEALTHY GUM   CROSS-SECTION DISEASED GUM

Periodontitis - Destruction of the bone around your teeth.

When the bacterial irritation and destruction reaches your bone, and the bone begins to be destroyed, it is called **periodontitis. Gingivitis can frequently be reversed; periodontitis, unfortunately, can only be arrested and treated; the lost bone structure often cannot be rebuilt.** In certain situations, lost structure can be rebuilt with bone grafts or special materials which, applied to the damaged area, allow gum and bone to regrow.

You may not recognize the change from gingivitis to periodontitis. It is gradual. You may see occasional gum bleeding that stops when you brush more. So you think you stopped the problem, but underneath the gum, you are continually losing bone. You may not think you have a problem until the teeth get loose. Then it is often too late. Sometimes the general dentist can treat this problem. Other times you are referred to a specialist called a periodontist. His practice is limited to periodontics, and he only treats people who have gum and bone problems and/or loose teeth. His intense focus on these tissues makes him uniquely trained among dentists to recognize not just the earliest stages of disease of the gum and bone, but to save teeth that otherwise might be extracted. Both the specialist and the general dentist who is periodontally trained can treat you and help you prevent loss of more bone structure, and teach you how to prevent future gum disease.

What Medical Conditions Can Periodontal Disease Cause When Untreated?

Recent research has linked periodontal infection (as a chronic disease) to cardiovascular disease, via at least two possible pathways: inflammatory byproducts in the bloodstream (from gum disease) leading to direct damage to the coronary arterial lining, and periodontal bacteria directly invading the coronary lining leading to atherosclerosis. Periodontal bacteria have also been associated with underweight newborns, lung disease, brain disease, blood clots and strokes, diabetes 2, and joint diease

CHAPER TWO

FREQUENTLY ASKED QUESTIONS ABOUT THE GUMS

Why do my gums bleed?

Gums bleed when the gum lining has broken down, and is ulcerated. You may notice this when brushing, or eating fruit, or using a toothpick or dental floss. If you follow proper plaque-control methods, or use water irrigation, you can stop the bleeding within a few days. If the bleeding is not stopped, periodontal disease gets worse, bone is lost around the teeth, and you may finally lose teeth.

If your gums happen to bleed spontaneously, without your even touching them, visit a dentist or physician immediately. A complete blood count should be taken to see if there is anything wrong with the cells of your blood. Certain conditions, such as leukemia, frequently show up first in the gum. Diabetes often shows up with early changes in the gums and bone, with abscesses, and bone loss. Your physician can help you by utilizing a fasting glucose test and another very important test, called HbA1C, to determine if you have diabetes.

What causes gum recession?

Gum recession generally is caused by excessive brushing, which literally "skins" the gum off the neck of the teeth. It can also be caused genetically, when the actual gum collar around the neck of the tooth is too short in height. This in turn allows the muscle fibers of the mucous membrane to pull at the gum border during lip and cheek movement, leading over time to gum recession. Sometimes orthodontic movement of teeth thins the bone near the gum margin so much that the bone dissolves causing the gum to then shrink to the new reduced bone level. Lastly, the gum may be receded because of prior periodontal surgery. Today, periodontists prefer to do surgical "flaps" to preserve the gum and clean underneath.

How can your gum recession be repaired?

There are several procedures used today, mainly by surgically trained periodontists, to cover over roots that have had recession. Your problem may require a special solution, and sometimes the gum can't be totally returned to where it was at age fifteen. Nevertheless, it can frequently be improved.

What happens if gum recession isn't treated?

The answer depends on several factors. For an older person, it might not be significant. For a younger person, or one in midlife, failure to correct an inadequate zone of gum where recession has already occurred can lead to further recession, gum irritation, and root sensitivity, and possibly also contribute indirectly to root decay or bone loss, and perhaps tooth loss.

What's the best kind of toothbrush?

For most people, a three- to four-row **soft** nylon brush with **rounded bristles** is best. It permits you to brush in the gum space correctly. It can be simple or electric or ultrasonic.

Is a Waterpik or any other kind of water irrigator important?

Water irrigators can be extremely helpful, and may help flush out food debris, loosen bacteria, reduce the bacterial count, reduce the biofilm layer, and flush dead cells from between the teeth and in the gum space. The technique used properly with flossing and brushing, produces excellent benefits. If a person is not really good with flossing, then using the water irrigator (Waterpik or other devices) is absolutely essential!

How often should I have my teeth cleaned?

This varies from patient to patient. Some people have greater susceptibility to gum breakdown. Others smoke, or drink more coffee or tea. Some people, especially diabetics, may form tartar more quickly. For an adult, about once every three months could be used as an average figure, especially if you have had periodontal breakdown. If you're very good with your mouth hygiene, you might only require it once every six months. You and your dentist should decide together, based on your dental history and personal plaque control efforts. Also, a tray system made at your dental office called PerioProtect is very helpful in controlling biofilm.

How does my diet affect my teeth? Are any foods especially bad?

Diet can affect your teeth greatly. Foods that contain sugar are particularly harmful, and the more concentrated the sugar the greater the danger. For example, caramels are worse than soda, and soda is much worse than freshly squeezed orange juice. Since sugar has also been indicted as a very probable contributor to diabetes, heart disease, and overweight problems, a careful person would do well to avoid sugar. Other foods that are not considered good for teeth are refined carbohydrates like gummy balls, potato chips, cookies, and pretzels. These also may lead to cavities, because the carbohydrate is attacked by bacteria on the teeth and converted to acids, which cause the teeth to decay.

CHAPTER THREE

EARLY TREATMENT OF GUM DISEASE AND BAD BREATH

The Cause of Gum Disease

We said earlier that plaque is a sticky transparent film composed almost entirely of colonies of bacteria. It also contains small amounts of cells, debris, and saliva. Plaque grows on the tooth above and below the visible gum line.

Since plaque can harden into tartar if not removed within twenty-four to thirty-six hours, it is most important for you to remove your plaque daily. Once it has hardened, you no longer can remove it; the dentist or dental hygienist has to do it for you.

For *this reason, it is most important for tartar to be removed at least every three months by a professionally trained person (a dentist, a periodontist, or a hygienist). If you keep your teeth extremely clean, you may only need a professional scaling and root planing every six months.*

Let's look at the relationship of plaque, tartar, and the gum lining. We see that on top of the rough, hardened tartar (which is adhering to the tooth); we have the living layer of bacteria. It lies directly against the lining epithelial cells of the gum, irritating and ulcerating them.

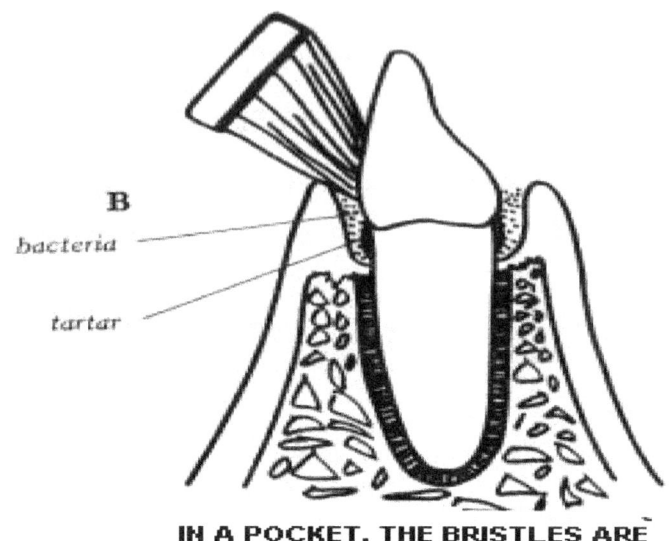

B

bacteria

tartar

**IN A POCKET, THE BRISTLES ARE
NOT FULLY ABLE TO REMOVE
THE BACTERIA**

Because of plaque's importance, you need to understand the following:

1. Organized plaque (the biofilm) is the enemy.
2. If not cleaned off, some of it hardens in thirty-six to forty-eight hours.
3. At that stage, you can no longer remove it, but must have it removed at the dental office.
4. After removal, it reforms in twenty-four hours to forty-eight hours.
5. On the surface of the tartar is still more living plaque, destroying your gum and bone.
6. If this process continues, as more bone is lost, teeth get loose, abscesses form, and must be removed.

GINGIVITIS: HOW TO REVERSE BLEEDING GUMS YOURSELF!

If you suspect that you have a gum problem, start taking better care of them. This can be done by brushing and flossing correctly, using a plastic toothpick in a special way, and perhaps a water irrigator. Your **dentist, periodontist or hygienist** will teach you how.

In addition, ask your dentist to "probe" your gums with a periodontal probe. This is a small measuring instrument that slips into the gum space between tooth and gum lining. It is marked in millimeters, and as the dentist measures on several sides of the tooth, he can assess how much gum detachment or bone loss has occurred. Probing is essential. Dental X-rays cannot show the amount of bone loss that the probe makes evident. Every tooth should be measured this way. Bleeding points and pocket depth tell the dentist if you have a problem.

PERIODONTAL PROBE

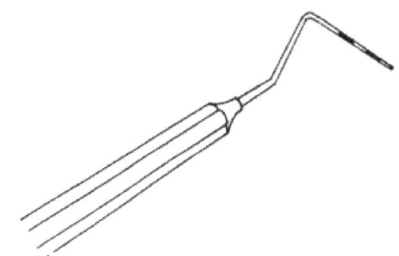

It has been shown that gum inflammation is directly related to poor oral hygiene. It can be reversed by daily removal of plaque. It must be daily because the bacteria completely re-form every twenty-four hours. If plaque is not removed within twenty-four to forty-eight hours, it starts to harden. Then, you can't remove it, and a dentist or hygienist has to remove the tartar. If it is not removed, it serves as a breeding ground for more bacteria. This leads to more breakdown.

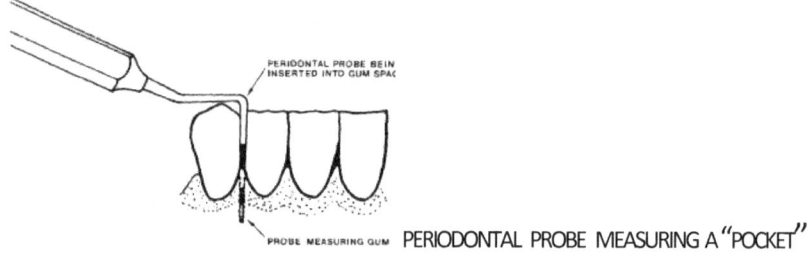

PERIODONTAL PROBE MEASURING A "POCKET"

CHAPTER FOUR

THE CAUSE OF TOOTH DECAY, BAD BREATH, BLEEDING GUMS, AND PERIODONTAL DISEASE

Remember one thing: Plaque doesn't only cause tooth decay and gum disease; it is the primary cause of bad breath. The odor comes from decomposing food and decomposing tissue and bacteria. Bad breath has been blamed on many things, from upset stomachs to garlic, onions, certain cheeses, milk, and smoking. All of these can increase the bad breath you already have.

But the single most important cause of bad breath is the food and bacterial plaque on your teeth and in the gum space, the decomposition of diseased teeth and gum tissue, and the coating on the surface of your tongue. If you remove plaque once a day, clean the top of your tongue, and have decayed teeth cleaned and repaired, most of your bad breath will be eliminated. Get those tender, bleeding gums, and gums with periodontal pockets fixed up, and you'll really start to smell kissable. As the advertising industry would say, "Keep the teeth and gums healthy, remove the plaque daily, and you'll be more desirable! Your mouth will feel clean and your breath taste fresh!"

Smoking will make it harder to have clean teeth and non-bleeding gums, because smoke stains leave rough surfaces on the tooth, which bacteria stick to. More bacteria, more odor. If you'd rather not offend anyone after eating, do the plaque control, and make sure, by being thoroughly examined by a careful dentist, that you have no dental disease.

Points to Remember

As we said earlier, although gingivitis is reversible, periodontal disease is not. As bone melts away from the gum infection, more bacteria get into the gum space, and more and more destruction occurs. As more bone is lost, the tooth may begin to get loose. At some point, pressures produced by normal chewing may actually rock the tooth in the bone. Continued rocking of the tooth loosens it still further, destroys bone, and may lead to your losing the tooth.

We know today that periodontal disease and tooth loss is not inevitable. It can be treated and the teeth saved. We know that gingivitis can be reversed. The key to this is early diagnosis and early treatment. And if you're young enough to still be periodontally healthy, then you can stay that way by removing the cause of early gum disease: bacterial plaque (biofilm), and keeping it away with PerioProtect trays.

Treatment of Gingivitis and Early Periodontal Disease

Gingivitis is treated by one or more visits to the dental office for thorough professional scaling and polishing of the teeth, and perhaps with procedures called root planing. This phase of treatment is frequently called initial preparation. It is the first stage of all periodontal treatment, and will allow the dentist to know whether or not you subsequently will require any surgical procedures. The word "cleaning" is a poor term. In some dentists' minds, it means scaling and polishing. To others, it means only polishing. The term "cleaning" should not be used, but when it is, think of it only as a polishing, or removal of visible plaque and stain above or at the gumline. Scaling would include removal of tartar. It may be done above the gum line only or extend into the gum space. The same is true for root planing, in which fine instruments are used to scrape and smooth the root surface to remove not only the tartar but also imbedded material and softened root structure. Root planing cleans the root under the gumline to the bottom of the gum space. It is often done under local anesthesia.

It is frequently most beneficial for you actually to be professionally taught plaque control, and then perform the plaque control first for several days before the professional cleaning, so you can actually see the change in your gum color and consistency. After four or five days, you will be amazed to see bleeding gums stop bleeding, tissues firm up, and redness turn to pink at the gum margin.

Periodontal Disease (Periodontitis)

The bone that surrounds and supports the tooth begins to be destroyed if the disease goes any deeper than the fiber attachment of the gum to the tooth. When the attachment is destroyed, and bone starts to melt away, the disease is called periodontal disease, or periodontitis. Pockets are now deeper and contain more destructive bacterial plaque. At this point, the condition is not reversible. Let's repeat that. Periodontal disease is not reversible. Now you have a problem. The problem is this: you are irreversibly losing bone! **Unfortunately, bone loss causes no pain until very late in the disease. This means that you could lose more than half your bone and not know it.**

There are some things you might see in looking at your own teeth and gums that would indicate possible bone breakdown.

- If the gums are shiny, swollen, or puffy, you may be losing bone underneath.

- If the gums have receded, and there are spaces in between your teeth, you probably have lost bone.

- If you have openings or spaces between teeth that you didn't have as a youngster, you probably have lost bone.

- Tooth looseness is another sign of advancing bone loss.

- You may also have bad breath.

CONTOUR OF NORMAL, RECEDED, AND INFLAMED GUM

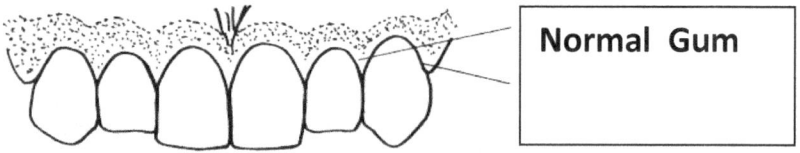

Normal Gum

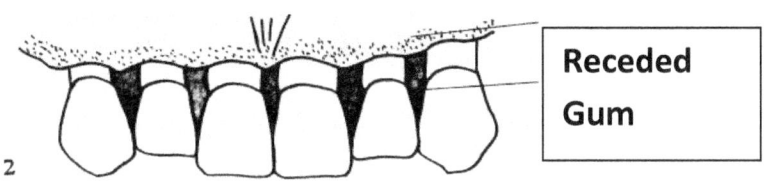

Receded Gum

2

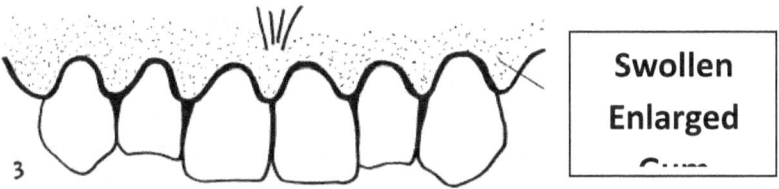

Swollen Enlarged

3

Points Worth Repeating:

- Plaque is the cause of both bacterial decay and gum disease.
- Plaque must be removed daily to slow or stop disease.
- Bacteria re-form in twenty-four hours. Therefore, you have to knock them out once every twenty-four hours.
- With proper mouth hygiene, and tartar removal at the dental office, gingivitis is reversible.
- Periodontal disease is not reversible, but is treatable. If not treated, you lose bone and later may lose teeth. It is a chronic disease that must be kept in balance by your efforts and periodic visits for professional tartar removal.

NOTE This mini-book will only concentrate on Periodontics, Implants, and Prosthodontics (mouth rebuilding). For greater detail regarding secrets of an attractive smile, pain control, dental insurance and the other dental specialties, you may want to buy the larger complete edition of this book called: "Dental Health & Treatment – Dental Cosmetics & Beauty" at www.infodentalhealth.com/sales.h

CHAPTER FIVE

HOW DECAY AND GUM DISEASE PROGRESS IN THE ADULT

Without bacteria your teeth would not decay. You have millions of bacteria in your mouth, mainly in cracks on top of your teeth, between your teeth, on teeth near the gum, and on the tongue. The bacteria have lunch on the food left on the teeth. As bacteria eat and digest the food left on the teeth, they form acids. These acids dissolve the hard mineral surface of your teeth and make holes. We call this process decay. We call the hole a cavity. Lots of holes equal lots of cavities.

The Tooth Decay Process

What plaque looks like under the microscope is shown in the illustration on page 8. There are some interesting facts to know about plaque and decay:

1. Studies have shown that without bacterial plaque, experimental animals on cavity-prone diets do not develop cavities.
2. Different bacteria are responsible for decay produced in different sites on the tooth.
3. Some bacteria cause decay on the sides of the teeth, some at the gum line, and others on the biting surfaces of the teeth. They work to destroy the enamel by forming acids.
4. As the acids and the bacteria get deeper into the tooth, different kinds of bacteria actually work together to destroy tooth structure.
5. Bacteria near the tooth surface need oxygen to live.

6. As decay progresses, other bacteria that require less oxygen take over in destroying the tooth.
7. Final result: Your hard tooth has a hole with soft rotting material in it.

The Role of Sugar

People and bacteria have something in common—they both love sweets! Some authorities believe that the worst sugar of all for teeth is sucrose, or ordinary white table sugar. Other authorities feel that glucose or fructose are pretty bad, too. Contrary to some people's belief, brown sugar is just as bad as white sugar. For generally good nutrition as well as controlling dental decay, cut those sugars as much as possible (glucose, fructose, and sucrose) (think of diet sodas, regular sodas, artificial sweeteners, etc) and refined carbohydrates (pastry). Refined carbohydrates are now also associated with diabetes 2. There are many modifying factors to the sugar-carbohydrate question, including:

8. The chemical structure of the carbohydrate eaten
9. Its consistency (solid, liquid, chewy, sticky, etc.)
10. When it is eaten (i.e., before bedtime, between meals, or with meals)
11. How free the mouth is from dental bacterial plaque when the food is eaten
12. How soon the mouth is cleansed after eating
13. The amount of fluoride in the enamel of the tooth
14. The acidity of the saliva (pH), and the acidity on the tooth from the food.

Surprisingly, small amounts of sugar are all that is needed to offer fermentable food to bacteria. Above those levels, additional carbohydrates or sugars do not seem to change the picture. Thus, in spite of current food fad mythology, the sugar-decay picture is not as simple and clear-cut as one would like.

Still, there are enough scientific papers which have found the role of the "sugars" to be of concern in causing decay that **it would seem prudent to greatly reduce eating or drinking foods with sugar. Try to only eat those sweets as dessert**

once/week, and skip the sodas and diet sodas, and the sweetened cereals.

It is obvious that sugar is found in many foods, in addition to being eaten in raw form. There's plenty of sugar in many baby foods, and in many cold cereals. Naturally, there's lots in jelly, jam, pancake syrup, and candy. Sure it tastes good, but what a price the child, or you, may pay in money, time, and maybe pain at the dental office.

Where On The Tooth Does Decay Occur?

It is helpful to know on which surfaces of the teeth the

decay most frequently starts, and also which teeth are most subject to decay.

Decay generally occurs on the biting surfaces of rear teeth that have "tops," or broad, crushing "tables," as opposed to front teeth, which really have biting "edges."

Decay on these rear teeth occurs in the fissures (cracks), or the pits on these "tables."

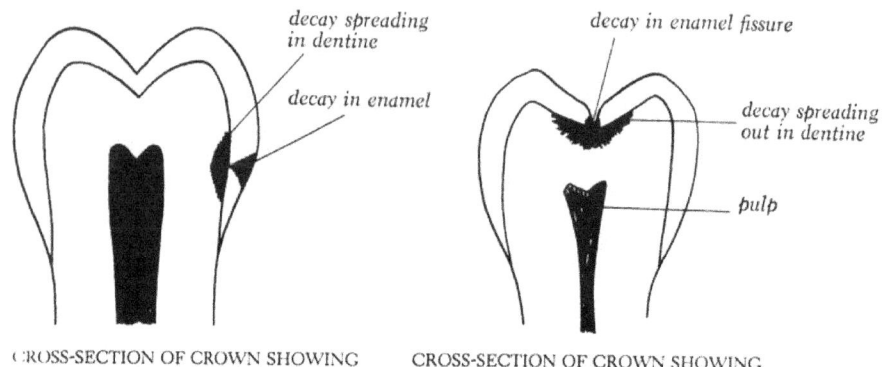

decay spreading in dentine

decay in enamel

decay in enamel fissure

decay spreading out in dentine

pulp

CROSS-SECTION OF CROWN SHOWING DECAY ON SIDE OF TOOTH

CROSS-SECTION OF CROWN SHOWING DECAY ON BITING SURFACE OF TOOTH

If you look at the top of your teeth in your mouth, you'll see grooves between solid areas of tooth structure. These are the pits or fissures. They can run very deeply downward through the enamel toward the dentine. They can look like the drawings in the cross section above. Beside the tops of the teeth, you can also get decay between teeth, just under the point where the teeth come into contact with each other.

Decay occurs in both the pit or fissure, and under the contact point, for two reasons: (1) food and bacteria collect easily there, and (2) they are tough places to reach with a toothbrush.

Lastly, decay can occur on the cheek or tongue side of the tooth next to the gum line. This most frequently occurs if the hygiene is poor. Decay also can occur under an old filling if the original decay was not totally removed. It can also occur if a new filling or gold inlay, onlay, or crown does not have fully sealed margins or edges next to the tooth enamel. Because hygiene plays such a major role in preventing decay, you should always brush and floss the entire tooth and gum line daily. Just because you've had new dental work, don't think that your teeth can't decay again. One of my patients thought that just because she spent a lot of time and money on her teeth, she had done everything necessary to have a healthy mouth. Not true! Poor dental hygiene means dental breakdown! Remember, just because a woman spends twenty-five dollars on a facial, that doesn't mean that she never has to wash her face again!

Deep Decay Can Cause a Nerve to Die

As the decay gets deeper into the dentine, the dentine decomposes, and gasses are produced by this dying material and by bacterial products. The gasses exert pressure on the nerve (pulp). You feel this as **a toothache**. The pain can be very intense. Remember, the pulp is surrounded on all sides by hard tooth structure. If infected or injured, some pulpal cells start to die, and other cells swell due to inflammation. The buildup of fluid and gasses in the pulp can cause swelling, which puts pressure on the tissue in the narrow opening at the root tip. With pressure from the inflamed nerve tissue, the blood supply to the pulp is restricted, or cut off. If this occurs, and the pulp dies, the nerves in the tooth can cause a great deal of pain as they undergo self-strangulation.

Saving the Tooth if the Nerve Dies

Do you have to lose your tooth if the nerve dies? The answer is no, whether you're an adult or a child. If a child has a toothache, the tooth may be saved, if not too badly decayed. This is done by taking your child to your dentist, or pedodontist (children's dentist). The tooth is anesthetized (made numb), and the dentist then cleans out the decay and removes the upper portion of the pulp where it enters into the root or roots. The procedure is called a pulpotomy. The adult gets a root canal filling after nerve removal.

When decay has not destroyed too much of the baby tooth, it is important to try to save it. It is important because it helps the permanent tooth to erupt into the proper space. If the tooth were extracted, the remaining teeth might crowd together to fill the space, and thereby block out the permanent tooth. These decisions are made by the dentist or pedodontist (children's dental specialist).

Decay in the Young Adult

The Twenties

From the twenties on, in addition to checking for cavities at the dental examination, we want to prevent decay to preserve the tooth and avoid nerve damage. Also, by twenty, a periodontal examination should be part of every dental examination. We want to stop periodontal disease as early as possible, because bone can't be replaced easily. It's much better to treat a patient in his twenties for early gum problems than to do extensive reconstructive periodontal surgery on a patient in his forties. The reason for this is that as more bone is lost, the surgical treatment gets increasingly complicated, and sometimes one has to remove roots, or teeth, or graft bone to rebuild the mouth. So this means surgery, healing time, and often substantial cost. So get a complete exam at the dentist including periodontal probing.

The Thirties— Dental Disease Is Now Taking Its Toll

The Missing Tooth.

By the time a person is in his thirties, several things may have happened. Some of you may have lost a tooth from decay in younger years. Or, if misadvised, you could also have lost one because you were told a tooth was beyond repair and you didn't get a second opinion. Lastly, you could have lost a tooth because during treatment, such as a root canal, something happened technically, making it impossible for the dentist to complete the root canal. You might have lost a tooth in an accident, or perhaps even missed one from birth. In any case, you now have a space or spaces in your mouth, and never bothered replacing the missing tooth or teeth because their absence never bothered you. Your appearance was O.K., and you seemed to chew adequately.

What you did not know was that there were shifts and changes occurring in the roots and supporting bone of the teeth adjacent to the space.

Shifting and Tilting, Causing Periodontal Destruction

Basically, what happens when you lose a tooth, particularly a rear tooth, is that the opposing tooth moves toward the space.

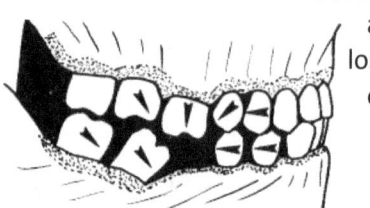

Seven teeth are affected and shift position by the loss of the lower first molar

Loss of the lower First Molar

This is particularly true of the missing lower first molar. The upper tooth drops into the space. Teeth next to the space lean in to try to fill it. There are actually seven teeth affected by the loss of the lower first molar.

Periodontal Destruction leads to tooth loss!

As these teeth shift and tilt, they no longer meet correctly while chewing. This puts extra pressure on the bone and periodontal ligament, causing a weakening in these supporting structures. If you have had your periodontal disease developing all along, when the disease reaches the areas of weakened bone and ligament, it progresses very rapidly and the periodontal pocket, with all its bacteria, gets much deeper. Ultimately, as the process accelerates, the deeper the pocket, the more pressure on the tooth from the unbalanced bite. This pressure can actually rock the tooth looser and looser. Finally, when the process has destroyed lots of bone, the tooth is so loose, or abscessing so frequently, that it has to be removed.

Therefore, losing the lower first molar can be like a chain reaction leading to many other problems.

If another tooth is lost from decay, or from an accident or periodontal disease, and not replaced, it too affects the position of the remaining teeth. As periodontal disease continues and more and more bone is lost, then teeth shift, are traumatized during chewing, become loose, and are eventually lost.

If your dentist does not examine you for periodontal problems, and merely suggests replacing the missing tooth with a removable or fixed appliance (like a fixed bridge, an implant, or partial denture) or the one visit inlay bridge called Bond-A-Bridge to be released in 2016 to dentists for patients, be concerned. You can't build a mansion on a swamp; you can't build a good bridge on a weak periodontal support, nor should implants be considered until the mouth is periodontally cleaned up. So get a good periodontal examination from a properly trained professional.

CHAPTER SIX

GOOD DENTAL EXAMINATION INCLUDES THE FOLLOWING:

1. Soft tissue, face and neck exam— FOR CANCER outside the mouth
2. Soft-tissue exam FOR CANCER inside the mouth
3. Examination of the jaw joint (TMJ) and chewing muscles for soreness.
4. Bite exam – Examination of how the teeth meet, chew, and slide.
5. Periodontal exam with pocket measuring and recording
6. X-ray examination showing crowns of teeth, the bone, and the tips of all roots.
7. Cavity check with clear visibility between teeth on X-Rays and mouth exam.
8. The consultation, summing up all the above information, with treatment and recommendations, including alternative choices.

Your dentist should explain what you need, why you need it, what the cost will be, and what choices you have. If you've never had this type of thorough examination before, you'll learn a great deal. Hopefully, after reading this mini-book, you should be able to ask some pretty intelligent questions, and get satisfactory answers.

Importance of the Periodontal Examination

The worst mistake you can make is not to get a thorough periodontal examination before undergoing restorative dental treatment as an adult. Restorative treatment may range from anything as simple as fillings, to more complex work such as inlays, onlays, or crowns.

Importance of Pocket Depth

At your regular "cleaning visit" (scaling and polishing), when your dentist measures your gum spaces with a periodontal probe, if your pockets measure deeper than 3 mm, your dentist or periodontist must decide whether the pockets can be controlled with further root planing and curettage or whether you need surgery. You should have antibiotic treatment for one week before the next root planning. Either the dentist or the periodontist may feel that the tissue will not benefit any more from conservative dental treatments (such as curettage or root planing). At that point, you will need to get those gum pockets reduced via a surgical trimming of the diseased gum wall and perhaps corrective or regenerative procedures to rebuild bone. Some periodontists may prefer to use an antibiotic product that is placed directly into the gum pocket for further shrinkage before moving on to surgery. In addition many dentists and periodontists will recommend special mouth washes or water irrigating devices. Another method being used now is to put a medicated gel into a closely fitting tray that goes over the gum and onto the teeth and pushes the medicated gel into the gum pocket. (PerioProtect

System) which is quite effective when used 2X/day. Recommendations are up to the particular clinician.

The primary purpose of all these treatment approaches is to create a shallow gum space after treatment that you can easily keep clean! Sometimes your periodontist or dentist might suggest you use baking soda, peroxide, and medicinal irrigation, to reach the full depth of shallow gum pockets rather than using surgery. Periodic visits and clinical observations plus probing will tell the periodontist or dentist if this method is working. If not, surgery will be indicated. For deeper pockets, surgery with pocket elimination is still the tried and true best method for eliminating the past tissue breakdown caused by the disease, according to most dental and periodontal authorities. **However, surgery alone is not the final answer. If you do not do plaque control daily, use an anti-bacterial rinse, or the trays with medicated gel, and go to the dentist for 2-4 visits a year for scaling and root planing, you will not keep the result that you achieved through surgery.**

CHAPTER SEVEN

WHAT KINDS OF TREATMENT ARE BEST FOR YOUR MOUTH

(Based on levels of severity of your periodontal condition and number of missing teeth)

Correct Sequence of Dental Treatment

Very important. If you do need periodontal treatment, it should always be done **before** the restorative dentistry, because your gum line is often further up the tooth after your periodontal treatment. It is impossible for a dentist or periodontist to treat the gums surgically after restorative dentistry without opening spaces between teeth. The new dental work must relate to the new gum line. The margin, or edge, of the new dental work should be gently placed either just into the new, healthy gum space, or a good bit away from it. If periodontal treatment does create spaces between teeth and restorative dentistry follows, then there is an opportunity to close some of those spaces. That is not possible when treatment is backwards, i.e., doing permanent dental work first and then, within a few years, following with periodontal treatment because of gum problems.

In a very comprehensive case, before any periodontal treatment is begun, it is a good idea for the dentist and periodontist to decide on one or two treatment plans for complete treatment. These plans must consider your financial ability to pay for your needed treatment.

You may find that the initial treatment plan is too costly. This sometimes happens. Ask the dentist for one or two alternate plans, costing less, that would still attend to your most important needs. Also ask him if he were to proceed more slowly with the ideal treatment plan, how long it would take to complete treating your mouth. Now consider each of the three possibilities, in terms of long-term value and cost:

1. Ideal treatment plan done within one year (may include implants and or bridge work).
2. Ideal treatment done over two or three years.
3. Alternate plan—less costly approach such as more frequent root planings and extraction of teeth with very deep pockets. It may also require removable tooth replacement appliances rather than implants or fixed bridge work. PerioProtect system would help.

List on a piece of paper the advantages or disadvantages of each. Narrow down to your two best choices. If you have more questions at that point, recheck with the dentist. Then go to the best person of your choice and get started.

If for any reason you cannot afford any plan, seek a second opinion. If it confirms the first opinion and you can't afford a private dentist, then your other financial alternatives would be to go either to a dental university or a hospital clinic near you. If you've listened carefully to the dentist's diagnosis and recommendations, ask the dentist for a copy of his recommendations. Using the written dental recommendations, you will know, if you go to a university or clinic, whether you are getting treated properly. Costs will be less there, but the work may not be as well done by the students or young graduates as they would be by an experienced dentist and/ or periodontal specialist. Obviously, you will spend much more time at a clinic or university than at a private office. So you must decide what your time and inconvenience is worth as opposed to the cost saving. Then you do whichever is better for your circumstances.

Two final recommendations:

First, if the dentist you are going to, or are thinking of going to, does not stress disease prevention, including plaque control and diet evaluation, or if you continue to have lots of decay, loosening teeth, or bleeding gums, look elsewhere. He's practicing in the past, not the present.

Second, beware of the dentist who claims he can do everything well. There are a few very highly trained dentists who are brilliant, both diagnostically and technically, but they are very rare. Most dentists are not doubly trained. Better to use a dentist and periodontal specialist unless the dentist tells you he has had a lot of periodontal training.

Therefore, if you have a periodontal condition that is moderate to severe (pockets of 6 to 9 mm), get to a good periodontist, a specialist in gum and bone treatment. If you need root canal work, and your dentist has done a lot of root canals, he would be fine for your problems. But if you don't think he's sufficiently experienced, consider seeing a root-canal specialist (endodontist). If your dentist wildly resists you going for second opinions, gets defensive, or feels threatened, chances are that he's not that confident of his diagnostic or technical abilities. He should respect your feelings and desire to make the right decision. Your relationship with your dentist is usually a long-term one. You both want to be comfortable with each other. Talk to him about your feelings, what you hope to get from his office, and his dental care, why you want to prevent disease and be helped in that direction. Give him a chance to cooperate and to grow with you.

If you find that he's uncooperative, defensive, or says that preventing disease is nonsense (and that tooth loss is inevitable), then get out fast! Do not walk, but run, to someone more current with today's knowledge, and who is more open-minded.

CHAPTER EIGHT

BENEFITS OF EARLY PERIODONTAL TREATMENT

Remember this: Although periodontal treatment can stop bone loss, and help save many teeth, it still cannot easily replace lost structure. Today we graft bone to rebuild some of the lost bone, and transplant gum to restructure tissues in ways we couldn't have clearly envisioned ten years ago. The next ten years will most likely introduce even more exciting and hopeful ways to rebuild lost structure. But these procedures may be costly, possibly painful, and take time. Frequently more extensive dental rebuilding is necessary in a mouth that has undergone periodontal destruction. We have no magic wand to wave to reverse things. And there is no magic mouthwash to use (yet) to eliminate plaque. So please be aware: the earlier you have your mouth probed and the earlier you are treated, the less extensive will be your ultimate therapy, and the less expensive will be your costs. In either case, to maintain your results after periodontal therapy, you still will have to do plaque control at home with flossing, brushing, water irrigating, rinsing with Chlorhexidine (Peridex) or similar antibacterial rinses, using trays with medicated gel twice/day, and gum compression. It's the only known way to prevent return of the disease.

Why Have Periodontal Surgery?

There has been a great deal of discussion among periodontists, and even in the public media, as to whether periodontal surgery is necessary, when it is, and why. We will expand on the reasons for periodontal surgery later. For the moment, just remember a few facts:

- The two causes of inflammatory periodontal disease are bacterial plaque and your body's hypersensitive reaction to material on the teeth next to the gum tissue.
- Since the toothbrush bristle and dental floss can get down into the gum space only about 3 mm (a little more than one eighth of an inch), once the gum space is too deep, the disease keeps going on unchecked! This deep gum space is called a pocket and it frequently harbors gum-detaching, bone-destroying bacteria, which brush and floss can't reach, nor can irrigating solutions.
- Special trays with medicated gels is the new long term solution after reducing pockets.
- And pockets must either be professionally cleaned out by the dentist or hygienist every 3 months, or periodontal surgery must be done to eliminate the pockets.

STUDY THESE DRAWINGS BELOW

gum space getting to the bottom of the space, which is shallow.
The drawing on the right shows the bristles do not get to the bottom of
the space in a diseased pocket. Further down are gum- and bone-
destroying bacteria, which, because they are not removed by brushing,
continue to do further damage

**The Below drawing shows bristles
being placed properly in a healthy
gum space getting to the bottom of the space, which is shallow.
The drawing on the right shows the bristles do not get to the
bottom of the space in a diseased pocket. Further
down are gum- and bone- destroying bacteria, which, because
they are not removed by brushing, continue to do further
damage.**

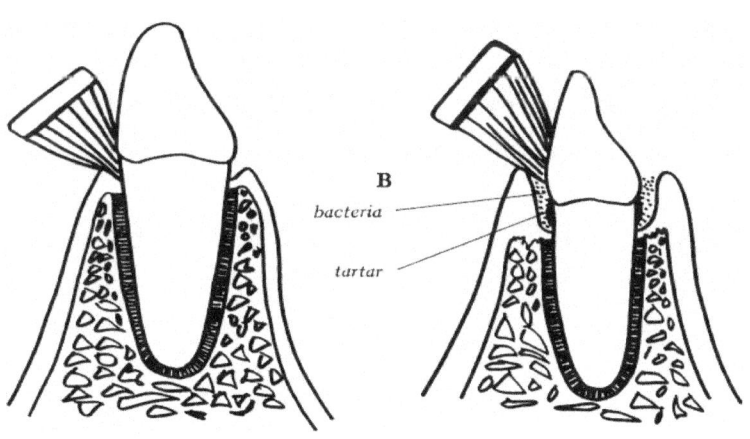

The reason some periodontal surgery is needed when the tissue is firm and the pocket measures 4-5 mm or beyond is that you cannot clean to the bottom of the gum space with floss, brush, or irrigation using salt solutions or medicinal solutions when the space gets too deep. There are frequently hidden depressions in the root contours at those pocket depths that are inaccessible to any cleansing by the patient. These areas harbor and breed bacteria. An older but critically important study in April 1978 by Waerhaug showed that beyond 3mm, the most meticulous root planing (scraping and smoothing the root surface clean of tartar and bacteria) failed to leave the tooth surface next to the pocket free of tartar and bacteria. Furthermore, the study showed that the deeper the pocket, the less possible it became to eliminate the harmful plaque and deposits. Only by reducing the depth of the pocket can we make those areas accessible, and also encourage a change from the more harmful type of bacteria to the less harmful type living in shallower gum spaces. Nothing has changed about this fact in over thirty seven years. After periodontal treatment, the medicated gel system (PerioProtect) is very helpful if used twice daily to keep the results.

CHAPTER NINE

PERIODONTAL TREATMENT – EVERYTHING YOU NEED TO KNOW

After initial scaling and hygiene instruction and allowing a few days to weeks of shrinkage and healing of the gums, when the dentist or periodontist again measures the pocket and finds the probe goes too deeply (4 mm or more), or finds that there is still some bleeding coming from the base or lining of the pocket, he knows he must treat the diseased gum more completely. Usually this means that periodontal surgery is necessary.

What Types of Periodontal Surgery Are Used Today?

Most periodontal surgery today consists of laying back the gum (like a flap) using local anesthesia. This reveals the underlying root and bone structure. Then the periodontist removes the results of past periodontal disease on the root and bone. As the gum flap is laid back, part of the diseased inner lining of the gum is also removed. With direct vision, all visible tartar still remaining on the root is removed, and the roots are planed smooth to remove deeply embedded bacterial debris. The bone is treated by removing the diseased tissue found at the bone crest, and then the shape of the bone is examined. There are certain anatomic requirements for the healthy bone that the periodontist sculpts and recontours into the damaged bone crest.

At times, when too much bone has been lost, the periodontist builds new bone. Bone grafting is the procedure used to build up missing bone. There are various ways to obtain the donor bone. Today, sterilized bone graft material is purchased from various companies by the dentist or periodontist. Some bone substitutes are totally synthetic and others are from human deceased donors who had no medical problems. When this material is used, it is sterilized, irradiated, and then treated with a strong acid, and absolutely purified. The bone is tested to make sure it is totally sterile. The sterilized bone has been ground to a fine particle size and used to enhance the formation of new bone. These materials come doubly sealed in glass bottles to the periodontist.

The success of bone grafting varies, depending on the area chosen, the type of defect into which the graft is placed, the periodontist's technical skills, and certain variables not controllable by the periodontist or patient. For example, teeth that have been exposed to periodontal disease for a long period of time (decades) may have a more contaminated root surface, which prevents the graft from forming a living connection to it. This cannot be determined in advance. Bone grafts, when correctly done in the properly chosen defect, work in at least 90 percent of cases. They are often well worth doing. Sometimes, even if the defect, after healing, is not totally refilled with bone, it is partially filled and one may then go back later and either regraft or contour the bone. Bone grafting and bone regeneration is one of our most exciting and hopeful areas in periodontics.

New Methods of Bone Regeneration – Tissue Engineering

Most recently, the field of tissue engineering, and stem cell research, has given us new tools with which to regenerate bone. One of the newest methods utilizes molecular extracts along the pathway of development from the basic mesenchymal cell. These growth factors have in turn been incorporated into a special vehicle which comes in a liquid form and is mixed with a powder that uses tricalcium phosphate chips. The material is placed directly into a bone socket after a tooth has been extracted. If the surgeon is growing bone on the floor of the sinus, then the bone cement is placed under the sinus membrane with a very small lateral opening in the bone of the upper ridge at the level of the sinus floor in order to provide enough bone to place implants. The amazing thing about the new technique is that the bone sets hard within a few minutes. This allows placement of implants immediately at the time of this surgery instead of having to wait anywhere from

3- 8 months before implants can be placed. The benefit to you is that you can have your final crowns placed on implants many months earlier than has been the tradition so far.

What Other Methods Exist For Treating Bony Pockets, such as Antibiotics or Special Rinses?

Combinations of antibiotic therapy may be used for short periods of time to reduce gum inflammation in conjunction with subgingival scaling and root planing. Some years ago, there were reports (by Dr. Paul Keyes) that using a saturated solution of table salt or baking soda to irrigate the gum spaces was helpful in controlling the harmful bacteria. Usually, a water-irrigating device (like the Water-Pik) or WaterFlossr, is used to squirt the solution into the gum space under low pressure. Today, different clinicians also recommend other medications that can be added to the reservoir container of the irrigating device. This solution is then pumped into the diseased gum tissues. Some clinicians have reported very good results, particularly for patients who cannot or will not undergo surgical procedures. Most clinicians feel that each patient has to be treated as an individual, and different mouths may require a combination of therapeutic approaches.

Chlorhexidine mouthwashes (Peridex is one example) have been successfully used to prevent plaque formation, and are very helpful in long term management of patients susceptible to periodontal disease. They require a dental prescription in the US.

Dental trays worn twice/day (PerioProtectSystem) with a medicated gel which squeezes into the gum space has now shown excellent long term results to control bacterial regrowth.

What if I have Diabetes?

You should get a blood test called an HbA1c to determine if you are pre-diabetic or outright diabetic, and your physician should medicate you depending on your test results.

How Long Does Periodontal Treatment Take?

Treatment can take as little as eight weeks, and as long as two years if orthodontics is involved. Most cases average between three and six months.

How About Pain?

This will vary greatly, depending on many factors. Your own pain threshold (i.e., how you interpret pain) is one of the biggest variables. The operator's skill, sterile environment, neatness, and quickness of opening and closing the wound make a difference. Your periodontal surgical procedures may be done in quadrants, half mouths, or as an entire mouth. Regardless of which approach is used, once you have been given local anesthesia (better known as Novocain or "shots") you will be completely numb and will not feel anything during the procedure. You should expect to use some medication to eliminate any pain that may occur after the anesthesia wears off. Your periodontist or dentist certainly will be able to provide you with a prescription to minimize any discomfort you will have.

In recent years, a small but growing number of periodontists have elected to do all the periodontal surgery in one or two visits so that you, the patient, will not have to experience surgical procedures repeatedly. Some people have assumed that if all sections of the mouth are done at once, or as a half-mouth procedure, there may be much more pain than from doing one quarter of the mouth. Actually, this is not true. Because those periodontists doing full mouth surgery have perfected efficiencies both in their procedures and in their coordination with their surgical assistants, less time is needed to treat each area. Thus the wound is opened and closed more quickly. There is no sacrifice in the quality of the result, yet there is less post-operative pain than one would expect. It is a surgical truism that the less time a wound is open to the air—and in the mouth, to the saliva and bacteria—the less trauma there is to the tissues. The less trauma, the less pain.

Generally speaking, the larger the area done each time, up to and including the entire mouth being done in one visit, the less pain per area you will have, assuming quick closure of the operated area. Remember, once you have any pain, you're going to take medication for it anyway. The fewer the number of procedures done, the less frequently you will be taking pain killers and antibiotics, and eating soft foods while wearing a surgical dressing on your teeth. Therefore, full or half mouth surgery has the advantage of your mouth being completed in one or two visits with the least amount of total medication taken, in comparison to quadrant surgery

In addition, with full mouth surgery, you don't have to think about having surgery a second time!

There are some advantages to doing smaller surgical areas. There may be less pain, but not always. You can eat more normally on the other side of the mouth. You may lose less time from work on each visit, but by the time your entire mouth is finished, you will have lost more time totally. This is because you probably lose lots of time running back and forth to the dental office when you have the surgical procedures done sectionally. With full mouth surgery there are fewer visits. There may be less swelling from sectional surgery since you'll only swell on one side of your face, but swelling only lasts a few days in either case. In both situations, there may be some slight leakage of blood for several hours. That is normal.

A word of advice: many periodontists place a dressing (bandage) that is like a thin rope of clay over the surgically treated gum area. Usually, bleeding stops within ten minutes, or sooner. If you have left the dental office, and are at home and find that you have bleeding or heavy leakage, use a wet 2" x 2" gauze pad, or a wet teabag and press the dressing for ten minutes, thus putting pressure on the gum under the dressing. It should stop the bleeding. Do not rinse for a few hours. If bleeding does not stop after trying this technique twice, call the periodontist.

Given the total variables involved in treating a moderate to severe periodontal condition, I feel that one or two surgical procedures is better accommodated by most people than the other method of doing the surgery in four or more visits. You have less fear and don't have to worry about having repeated surgeries. Sometimes if you require it, you will be sedated at the dental office, and this will also help to relax you. Only if medical, psychological, or age factors (like a slower healing response) weigh heavily would I suggest doing periodontal surgery in small sections. This is a personal preference based on my observations after years of doing periodontal surgery.

What About Sensitive Teeth After Periodontal Treatment?

It is true that initially you may experience sensitivity to heat and cold if you have roots exposed. This is usually temporary and tends to disappear between four and twelve months after periodontal treatment. Its removal may be facilitated by application of special solutions (stannous or sodium fluoride, other solutions, or adhesive resin applications painted onto the root surface by your dentist). Your own efforts at home, using Sensodyne toothpaste, also may help desensitize the teeth more rapidly. At times, when the teeth are in provisional (temporary) crowns or bridges, there is some sensitivity at the edge of the plastic crown.

The sensitivity may be reduced by recementing the crown or crowns or adding a little extra bonding plastic to cover the sensitive area. After surgery, some teeth that are unduly sensitive may need crowns, and occasionally root-canal treatment, if they cannot be adequately desensitized. Sometimes this type of tooth has greatly reduced bone support, and will be joined to its neighbors with additional crowns (splinting).

In summation, although sensitivity may occur in some mouths, your dentist or periodontist will be able to solve the problem over a period of a few months or less. Give him your patience and your cooperation.

Will I Need Extensive Dental Work After Periodontal Treatment?

You may or may not. It will depend on several factors. If you are missing teeth, you will need replacements. *If you are going to have a higher gum line on the front teeth, particularly the upper teeth, there will be some spacing between the roots, and it may show when you smile.* You may want to crown six or eight of the upper teeth, so that your smile and speech look and sound normal. For rear teeth, the decision as to whether or not to crown the teeth will depend on the degree of tooth looseness (periodontally involved teeth usually have some looseness to them). If extensive mobility persists after periodontal therapy, including bite adjustment, you may require gentle orthodontic rearrangement of the teeth to create a less traumatic bite, or you may need permanent splinting with crowns.

Frequently careful bite adjustment in which excess stresses on the teeth are removed by selectively grinding "high" or interfering surfaces, will reduce or eliminate tooth mobility. Slight mobility is acceptable and, if you are given a choice between cutting down and capping your teeth versus having slight mobility with a good prognosis, I would recommend slight mobility and not cutting down the teeth. Remember, I said slight mobility. Your periodontist should make the final decision on splinting, based on his evaluation of your teeth during treatment or at the completion of active treatment.

Frequently, on more complicated cases, several consultations are held with the restorative dentist, the periodontist, and you. At that time, an optimum plan is presented to you that will best protect the remaining teeth and their structures and/or replace missing teeth. Based on the professional recommendations and your budget, a course of treatment can be arrived at that will accomplish the most for your mouth and still stay within your financial means. You may consider implants as part of rebuilding lost teeth.

What Does Periodontal Treatment Cost?

The most important aspect of the fee is the value you place on retaining your teeth. If you save your teeth with professional help, then you will have saved a great deal of money also, since missing teeth are much more costly to replace than saving your own. The earlier you are treated, the greater the savings will be.

Assuming That I've Had Thorough Periodontal Treatment, Will It Last? Can I Still Lose My Teeth?

Generally speaking, with proper planning on the part of your periodontist, your dentist, and yourself, you should be able to retain all the treated teeth, if your professional team so advises you.

Sometimes the condition may be so advanced at the time you present yourself that no assurance can be given that all teeth can be saved. Hopeless teeth may have to be removed. If, however, you are treated early enough, and if you are taught plaque control and do it once daily, you should have a fine result. This assumes that you are in good health, with no diabetes or any other condition, which by itself, or as a result of treating the condition, weakens the gum or bone. You should also understand that since mouth bacteria are always present, as is the saliva with its mineral salts, you may still form tartar, with living bacteria on its surface. Therefore, *periodic visits to the periodontist and/or dentist approximately three months apart for professional scaling, root planing and polishing are necessary for the treated patient*. These are called *maintenance visits*. Again, long term, the PerioProtect system has shown to control return of the bacteria. Frequent probing should continue to be done, as a relapse in a specific area may occasionally occur. If it does, by going to your dentist and/or periodontist frequently, he will detect the slightest early breakdown and be able to treat it easily.

Remember, you are the biggest variable. If you don't keep the bacteria away from the necks of the teeth daily, you are again susceptible to breakdown. If you do not see your periodontist or dentist frequently for subgingival root planing, you may have a return of periodontal disease. Do not be discouraged if you find that you are not disciplined enough to do plaque control daily. Just acknowledge it, tell your periodontist or dentist that you have a problem with always doing it, and ask him if you may come in more frequently for professional scalings. You can floss at night when you watch television to make it easier.

Years ago, studies in Sweden and the U.S., indicated that very frequent professional scalings will help control the disease even in a mouth that is not adequately maintained by the patient, or that has some shallow pockets. Therefore, there are two solutions to follow-up care. You control plaque once a day, use the medicated gel trays twice/day, and go in less frequently for professional scaling, root planing and reexamination (perhaps twice/year) OR, if you're not as good as you should be, then go in more frequently to see your periodontist or dentist and have your teeth professionally scaled. Based on current knowledge, and with this type of approach, you should retain your teeth for many more years. Add to this the use of water irrigation or PerioProtect trays, and you have the opportunity to keep your teeth, rather than get dentures in your later years. Your own teeth are much more comfortable than dentures. Your own teeth allow you to chew better, speak better, and give you the psychological comfort of knowing that when you go to sleep at night, part of your mouth (the denture) isn't floating in the glass on the night table!

CHAPTER TEN

THE DENTAL SPECIALTIES

There are eight specialties that are recognized by the American Dental Association. Of these, six are clinically important enough for you to know about. In addition, there is a discipline: *Implants,* which allows you to replace missing teeth. Although not formally recognized as a specialty, implants are so important we are going to discuss them here.

The six clinical specialties are:

PEDODONTICS—children's dentistry

PERIODONTICS—treating diseased gum and bone, and helping rebuild the dentally neglected mouth in conjunction with the dentist.

PROSTHODONTICS—repairing damaged teeth and mouths and replacing missing teeth and jaw structure

ORAL SURGERY—removing teeth and lesions of the soft and hard tissues of the mouth, repairing fractures, and surgical procedures in the head and neck area.

ENDODONTICS—root-canal treatment.by removal of the nerve of the tooth.

ORTHODONTICS—straightening teeth, guiding growth and development of the jaws

IMPLANTS (not officially a specialty)—placing formed structures onto or into the jawbone to help anchor tooth replacements firmly to the bone and oral tissues.

The Specialist

What is a specialist? He is a dentist who by virtue of special training, education, and exposure to other more knowledgeable specialists in a particular field, ultimately becomes expert in diagnosing and treating conditions in that field. Frequently this education is a formal two or three year training program. It may include special training in a hospital. It usually involves discussing complicated cases. The specialty schooling tries to cover all known information about problem conditions in that specialty and ways to solve those problems and return the patient to health. The specialist is trained to set the example in quality care for the rest of his profession in his particular discipline. He actively associates professionally with other specialists in his field, and thus stays very well informed of new developments in his own specialty. He frequently teaches, writes, and tries to share his knowledge with general dentists to inform them of these new developments.

Periodontics and the Periodontist

The Periodontist is a specialist trained to treat diseases of the gums and bone, and the supporting structures of the teeth. He has usually had two or three additional years of training beyond the four-year dental school curriculum. He is very well trained in Oral Medicine, as well as diagnosis of poor occlusion (how the upper and lower teeth meet), and how occlusion influences the jaw joint (TMJ). He is an expert in both helping prevent periodontal disease, and uses knowledge of oral microbiology in treating periodontal disease. He uses medical testing, and both non-surgical and surgical methods to obtain his results. Today he also uses bone regeneration techniques to regrow lost bone around the teeth and to regenerate bone where it is needed in order to place the implants.

He is also very well trained in placing implants.

Prosthodontics and the Prosthodontist

Prosthodontics is defined as "the art of making dental appliances and substitutes such as crowns, bridges, artificial dentures, etc." * Most dentists make the above dental replacements, but certain dentists have had special formalized prosthodontic training for two or three years beyond dental school. They have studied some of the most difficult problems that a dentist may face in rebuilding a mouth. When they complete the extra years of education, these dentists are called prosthodontists, and they join a very small, select group of specially trained dentists around the country.

Prosthodontists are frequently referred to as courts of last resort for rebuilding difficult mouths. They may be asked to treat very difficult denture patients, or patients who have great difficulty

* *Dorland's Illustrated Medical Dictionary* (Philadelphia: W. B. Saunders).

wearing removable appliances. They may be asked to design a stable replacement in a mouth that has very few teeth left, without rocking loose the remaining teeth. They frequently are involved in a service called *mouth reconstruction* (as are many well-trained dentists), usually in conjunction with a periodontist. Because of their special emphasis on creating a proper bite, creating the proper relationship of the jaws to each other, of the jaws to the temporomandibular joint, of the teeth to each other, and of the muscles of the lips and face to the teeth, they—as well as a dentist who has taken many courses in the above areas—are particularly equipped to treat difficult cases.

If you are a patient contemplating a full mouth reconstruction with a great deal of dentistry to be done, and trying to choose between a well-trained dentist and a prosthodontist, these are some logical questions you might ask. Has the general dentist had sufficient experience in full mouth rehabilitation, and does he feel that he can handle all the variables as well as they should be so you get the best result? How will you know, if the dentist says he can do it, that indeed he can? The only way to solve this problem is to ask the dentist if you might meet and talk with a few patients for whom he has done this kind of work, to see how they look and how comfortably they chew. Perhaps a more important question to ask is which periodontist he would like you to work with. If he says that he can do your periodontal work, I'd be very cautious if your mouth has had a lot of bone loss. I personally would not feel comfortable unless the dentist has had numerous courses in periodontics, during which he was able to get continuous, supervised clinical instruction and an opportunity to follow up his cases later on to see how they were doing. Periodontal treatment is very complicated, and very few general dentists today can obtain the same results a good periodontist can.

However, there are some dentists that have had extensive training in both. Therefore, I recommend that you go to a periodontist on your own, and get a second opinion from him on how bad your gum disease is, before a final decision..

You might also have an independent consultation with a prosthodontist, and ask him about the dentist wanting to do the mouth rehabilitation. There are many dentists who have the skill to execute it successfully, and many who don't know their own limitations. Since you may be spending tens of thousands of dollars on your mouth before you're finished, you really have an obligation to yourself to be with the right team.

In speaking with capable dentists and prosthodontists, I asked them what was paramount in a successful case. Their answers consistently referred to quality, higher standards, wanting better work from laboratories, sending the work back if it didn't meet their standards, and so on. The diagnosis of what each mouth required was another major point. Someone once said, "Many people hear, but few people listen!" Similarly, many dentists may "look," but few may really "see." The capable dentists and prosthodontists search for nuance and detail. They consider all aspects of a case. Their ability to know when a problem exists, how to solve it, and which peer to go to should they want to discuss an unusual case, all make for a better final result.

CHAPTER ELEVEN

(Usually Placed by a Periodontist, Oral Surgeon, or a Dentist well trained In Implant Placement)

The Endosseous Implant (in the Bone) (Root Form Implants)

The most commonly used type of implant today is the root implant. Prior to the implant placement procedure, X-ray analysis, often including CT scans, is done in order to determine the size and shape of the implant to be used for a particular site and to see if there is enough bone present. The implant must be placed into the bone where there is sufficient depth and thickness of bone remaining. It must avoid, when possible, penetrating the sinus, or hitting the mandibular nerve. Today, because of the success of bone grafting, and because often the bony ridge is sometimes not thick enough or high enough to place an implant, the periodontist or oral surgeon must first use bone grafts in order to build up adequate bone to place the implant. Additional X-rays and CT scans may need to be taken if bone grafting has been done before placement of implants. These final X-rays will determine the diameter and length of the implants to be placed.

The endosteal implant (root form) is placed by reflecting the gum tissue to expose the underlying bone. Holes are placed into the bone, and the implant is then partly screwed into position. Trial X-rays are taken during the procedure to make sure that the direction of the implant is correct. If everything is fine, the implant is screwed into its final position, and the gum is sutured closed.

The endosseous implant can be used in combination with

natural teeth, to replace missing teeth with a fixed bridge, or one may have several implants in a row with individual crowns on them, replacing several missing teeth.

Here are examples of the root portion of the implant to the left, and the implant with the post (abutment) illustrated on the right.

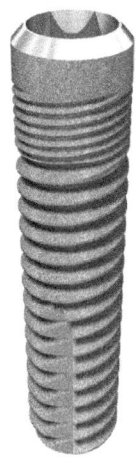 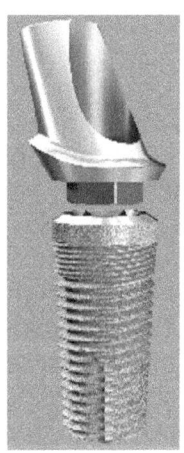

Placing several implants in a row often will permit making a dental replacement that is superior to a removable partial denture. Several implants have also been used occasionally to replace a lower denture in a person with adequate bone to support a denture, but who really hates taking the denture in and out of the mouth. In addition, another way that implants are being used successfully is to anchor full dentures so that they don't slip and slide around, making eating difficult. This is particularly true of the lower denture, where implants have proven to be extremely helpful.

A new addition to the implant field that has gained tremendous popularity for tightening loose dentures is the mini implant. This implant, because it is smaller in diameter, has been able to be placed without open surgery or with very little surgery into very narrow ridges, and can then be used to support the denture. They also can be used as an additional bridge support by placing the implant directly through the fixed bridge in the area of a false tooth. These mini implants have been tested now for quite a few years and are proving to be extremely helpful to patients.

It must be understood that with implants, as with all dental procedures, no guarantees can be given as to how long they'll last. Chances for your success are good if your health is good, and if you intend to be careful and attentive with your oral hygiene. It is a known fact that chronic smoking, as well as alcohol abuse, will shorten the longevity of implants.

After placement of the implant, your dentist should see you at very frequent intervals. He will advise you about the frequency of checkups. He wants to make sure that the implant isn't loose, that there is no infection or inflammation, and that the gum is healthy. You should be relatively comfortable when chewing in order to consider your implant successful. Again, for long term control of biofilm, the medicated trays of PerioProtect are helpful.

CHAPTER TWELVE

MOST FREQUENTLY ASKED ABOUT IMPLANTS

1. *What are the main advantages of root-shaped implants?*

Root implants provide a useful service for people who have difficulty with removable appliances. Whether the removable is a full denture or a partial denture, it is frequently uncomfortable and causes gagging for certain people. If you are one of those, you should investigate the possibility of root implants attached to the replacement teeth which are fixed and would remain in your mouth. It is important that the dentist, periodontist, or oral surgeon you choose for the implants be experienced in placing implants, and has a good reputation for the end result.

Successful implants provide extra chewing comfort and the psychological satisfaction of knowing that at night your bridges are not going to be removed and placed in a glass of water.

Implants are used today when teeth are periodontically weak, and need to be removed; when prior root canal work is failing and retreatment is not considered a good option, as well as to replace missing teeth. Your appearance and speech may be better with implants and reconstruction than with a denture. In addition, remaining bone support may be preserved longer (just as with real roots) than if your toothless jawbone had to support a denture.

2. *Are implants usually successful?*

Today most implants are successful if the initial diagnosis is carefully made and the patient is felt to be a good candidate, medically, anatomically and psychologically, to receive an implant. Again, the implants should be placed by an experienced practitioner. Even after 10 years, most implants are still in the bone and functioning well.

You might ask the dentist or surgeon how many implants he has done and how long he has been doing them.

3. *What are implants made of?*

Implants must be biocompatible, i.e., they must be inert in the tissues and not promote rejection mechanisms of the body. The most commonly used material is titanium. Sometimes the titanium is coated with hydroxyapatite, the crystal that enamel and bone are made of.

4. *Where are the root shaped implant procedures done?*

They are typically done in your surgeon-dentist's office during regular hours. Any discomfort following the procedure can be adequately handled by prescription medications given to you to get before the actual procedure. Some implant procedures may be completed in one visit; others may require two or three. In addition, there will be a certain number of dental visits to construct the replacement teeth which will fit on the implant. Often replacement teeth are ready at the time of implant placement so you walk out with teeth.

5. *Are implants costly?*

Cost is always relative. The cost of the mplants is relative to the community, city, state, country, and the skill level of the surgeon or dentist placing them. Often there are separate charges for bone grafting, or periodontal treatment. These can add to the cost, but must be done to get the right result. None of these costs refer to the prosthetic devices or crowns that will be fitted over the implants. The subperiosteal implant, which would include both the implant and the superstructure (teeth fitting onto the implant) will also range depending on what geographic community it is placed in, and the experience of the surgeon placing it.

6. *Who should not have implants?*

People with uncontrolled endocrine problems such as diabetes should not have implants unless the diabetes is well controlled. The same is true for any severe metabolic disorder or condition being treated with any medication that could affect the tissue or bone. Post-menopausal women with inadequate bone density may be taking medications like Fosamax or similar pharmaceuticals which could create major healing problems if implants were placed. Certain herbal formulas will prevent adequate clotting and cause prolonged bleeding, and should not be taken when implants are being placed.

You must advise the dental surgeon about any medication or herbs you are taking, or any allergy that you have. Generally, subject to a total review of your medical history by the surgeon and perhaps a consultation by him with your physician if necessary, any patient who can physically, emotionally, psychologically, and financially undergo bridgework and/or extractions could undergo dental implant procedures. Your individual dentist should help you make the right decision. Any remaining teeth should receive periodontal treatment before the implants are placed.

7. *What may I expect the day the implant is inserted?*
    Your gum tissue will be made numb, the same as for a routine filling. You may experience some soreness or tenderness following the implant placement after the anesthesia wears off. Mild pain relievers will take care of this discomfort. This is true of the root implant. If necessary, your dentist or surgeon will provide you with stronger pain pills if he feels they are indicated. The subperiosteal procedure may cause more discomfort and swelling, but this too is controlled with proper medication. Such swelling may last for a few days. Usually with a subperiosteal implant, the patient leaves the office with temporary teeth attached to, and sitting over, the implant. This is also true if you have root placed implants in the front of your mouth. You need not fear walking around toothless. Except for the implants in the front of your mouth, generally you will not walk out with temporary replacement teeth the same day, although with the use of surgical stents (guides for implant placement), some patients with adequate finances and enough bone are able to get their final teeth the same day implants are placed. You definitely will be able to eat soft foods, smile, and speak, even if your chewing requires a little compromise. A soft diet is recommended during this period. After a short period of time (a few days to a few weeks), eating will be more normal.

8. *When will the permanent teeth be put in?*
    Final teeth are placed within three to five months following

implant placement. That is after any bone regeneration procedures which themselves can take 4 to 7 months. The exception to this is the **immediate implant**. The past few years have brought evidence of increasing success in immediate placement of various prosthetic devices over implants on the same day. This is very expensive, but by taking special X-rays and using special dental laboratories, the dental prosthesis can be fabricated in advance of the surgery and placed at the time of surgery. It does require extreme exactitude on everybody's part, but the technology is here and is being done with great success for those that can afford it and whose dental condition lends itself to this approach. There are specific indications for doing immediate implants but they are not appropriate for most implant situations. Usually you are better of with a submerged implant, which will stay in the bone for 3 – 5 months until it locks to the bone and becomes immovable (integrates). After this time period, the post and later the crown may be placed. Each patient, as a unique human being, has his or her own particular variations and therefore your own mouth must be considered on an individual basis. Once replacement teeth are placed, there will be certain adjustments made for you by the dentist in adjusting your chewing comfort. Your dentist may have to adjust your bite a few times before you are comfortable. Eventually, you should enjoy the new stability with which you can eat. Remember that although the implant reconstruction may function much better than your old denture, it is still not like your normal teeth.

9. How *do I care for my teeth now?*

Your hygiene must be very good. Bacterial plaque forms around the teeth and the necks of the implants. You should remove plaque daily with flossing and brushing, and water irrigation and you should also have your teeth cleaned periodically by your dentist.

10. *What happens if the implant doesn't work out? How will I know, and what will I do?*

If the implant isn't working, it may get loose or it may hurt. Since you should be seeing your dentist regularly, he should see the problem and advise you. If necessary, a failing implant can be removed and in most cases replaced after a period of time is allowed for healing. There may be a need for some bone grafting before replacing an implant.

11. *How long can I expect the implant to last?*

Subperiosteal implants have an excellent track record. They have been in people's mouths as long as twenty-five years and more. Placed on a ridge with the proper type of bone support, and in a patient with a relatively normal medical history, their prognosis is very good. However, they are not used too much these days. Instead, root forms are used.

Root form implants have been used with success since the 1960s. They are considered successful when they last seven years and beyond. In the beginning they were used everywhere in the mouth, and for many purposes. Today, properly placed root form implants have had very high success rates (well over 90%) after ten years, depending on the type of prosthesis placed over the implants. They have been tremendously improved in design in the last ten years, and have been most successful where a decent number of well-supported natural teeth remain. When the entire case is supported by implants, it receives greater stress, therefore the denser the bone and the more implants that are placed, the stronger the case. Again, hygiene around the implants is extremely important to reduce tissue breakdown. Patients with a history of clenching, grinding, or bruxing their own teeth, and who continue to clench and grind with implants, are placing them (as well as any of their own remaining teeth) under greater stress. This may shorten the life of the implant. If the prosthesis is fixed bridgework, a patient that clenches or grinds his teeth should wear a nightguard. Patients with any history of uncontrolled diabetes or other health problem that retards healing and repair will find that the longevity of implants will be shorter.

With the above considerations respected, you should find implants of benefit to you,

CHAPTER THIRTEEN

OTHER FREQUENTLY ASKED DENTAL QUESTIONS

How often should I go to the dentist?

At least once every six months for a few X-rays, cavity check, probing, and cleaning. You would do better, on average, going four times a year, unless your dentist advises you that that frequency isn't necessary. Scalings and root planing on people over thirty should be done at least every three months, unless the patient is very good with plaque control. It would help if you were checked for periodontal disease or new breakdown by being re-probed with written records being kept, especially of bleeding points and pocket depth.

What causes me to grind my teeth at night?

Grinding may be the result of many factors. Most commonly, it is a manifestation of inner tension or aggression. Infants have been observed, even before teeth enter the mouth, to move their jaws in the same manner that adults do. The infant seems to be satisfying very basic needs of tension reduction by rubbing his lips and gum pads against each other. After teeth erupt, the habit of rubbing to reduce tension may continue, except now the teeth are rubbed against each other, rather than the gum pads.

Another reason for grinding described in the literature is a lack of harmony between upper and lower teeth meeting fully with each other, and their relationship to the jaw joints. This occurs when the patient attempts to close comfortably, and, not being able to, tries to position his jaw so that his teeth do not slip against each other. If his teeth are slightly out of exactly correct occlusion, his struggle to place them in a comfortable position causes him to keep searching for the most comfortable position with lower jaw movements. **This forward-and-back, or side-to-side movement, rubbing the teeth against each other, is called bruxing.**

Can bruxing cause damage?

Yes. Teeth can be worn excessively. Sometimes, the jaw joint may hurt, or the pain may be referred to the temples, side of the face, neck, or shoulders. Headaches may occur.

How is bruxism usually treated?

Most commonly, the dentist does a bite adjustment (spot-grinding on the biting surfaces of the teeth with a high speed bur) or a series of such adjustments, to eliminate obvious slips or interferences. This hardly removes any tooth structure at all and causes no pain. If opening of the jaws is limited, it is sometimes necessary to use a night guard or Hawley bite-plane appliance to break the muscle spasms preventing the jaw from fully opening. After wearing this appliance for several weeks, and sometimes taking a muscle relaxant or tranquilizer in addition, the jaws become sufficiently relaxed to allow for wider opening. At that point, the bite is again checked to eliminate any cusp interference or slips. These are eliminated by selectively grinding the proper marks on the teeth. It should be noted that generally the approach described is treating symptoms, not causes. Underlying tension or aggression may also have to be dealt with, possibly via psychotherapy.

What is a night guard?

A night guard is a thin piece of plastic specially formed to fit over your upper or lower teeth. It is worn at night while you sleep. Its purpose is to prevent you from grinding or clenching your own teeth, which could damage the teeth, roots, and supporting bone. When you wear the night guard, if you do grind (or brux your teeth at night), you only damage the surface of the night guard. One type of night guard that only fits over the front teeth has been introduced successfully in the past 15 years. It is called the "NTI" and is very effective with the right dental situation. It is smaller than the usual night guards, and is worn on the upper or lower front teeth.

Why is a tooth sometimes sore after a new filling or crown is placed?

This can be due to the fact that the filling or crown is "high." This means that there is excess dental material preventing the opposite tooth from closing down completely on the newly restored tooth when the jaw closes. Treatment would be to adjust the bite on the newly restored tooth and the opposing one until all bite marks on the teeth are in proper position, and the patient is comfortable. This can happen with fixed bridgework, partials or full dentures,

What causes a "toothache"?

A toothache can be caused by deep decay; by a periodontal pocket; by a fracture or vertical split in the tooth; by an incorrect biting relationship between that tooth and the opposing one; and by trapped gas under an old filling or crown. Sometimes teeth that have received a white bonded filling get sensitive. This is usually a technical issue and the filling must be removed and replaced within the first two weeks, usually with a desensitizing primer and adhesive liquid before placement of the new white filling. If too much time goes by before the new filling is placed, the tooth may require a root canal. Sensitivity is often caused when either the tooth enamel or the covering of the root (the cementum) has been worn through, and the dentine is exposed. Dentine is much more sensitive to heat and cold than the enamel or cementum, and stimulation from heat or cold is experienced as pain or ache.

As described above, a tooth can be sore if the dental replacement is "high" when chewing against the opposite tooth. The dentist must quickly adjust this.

My teeth are sensitive at the gumline. Can anything be done about this?

There are several approaches used today. One approach, when possible, is to add a dental material called resin to the sensitive root area and cover the sensitive roots. A second approach is for your dentist to use one of several available materials (either fluoride or calcium hydroxide derivatives) on the sensitive root areas, and repeat this procedure several times. This stimulates the nerve to lay down more tooth structure to insulate itself from temperature changes. Certain toothpastes are designed to decrease sensitivity over time.

What are the chances of having periodontal disease?

You are almost guaranteed, if you live long enough, to develop periodontal disease, but there is hope that you can avoid it if you read and apply carefully the information in this mini book, and what you are taught by the dentist and /or hygienist regarding controlling plaque with proper brushing, flossing, use of water irrigators, and the twice/day PerioProtect system..

CONCLUSION

I hope this book has been helpful to you and perhaps your family in understanding more about where dental disease comes from, how to replace your missing teeth, how to have any gum problems or loose teeth taken care of, helping you to perhaps use your dentist or dental team wisely, and most importantly taking some of the fear out of dental unknowns by giving you the information to help you make better dental decisions.

Sincerely,

Dr. Howard Marshall

PS. Should you be interested in more complete information to help your children or to help you with dental information during a pregnancy, or more information about regular dentistry such as fillings, inlays, onlays, crowns, fixed bridges, white fillings, bleaching, veneers, orthodontics (braces), Invisalign, children's dentistry, saving money on dental costs, and dental insurance, you might consider the larger book that preceded this book. It is called "Dental health & Treatment – Dental Cosmetics & Beauty". You can find this on Amazon.com. You can also purchase it as a download at http://www.infodentalhealth.com.

NOTE: FOR DENTISTS AND DENTAL OFFICES THAT WISH TO GIVE THEIR

PATIENTS COPIES OF THIS BOOK, IT IS AVAILABLE AT BULK DISCOUNT

BY CONTACTING DR. MARSHALL VIA EMAIL AT: ddshelps@yahoo.com

Cost for 12 copies or more will be $5.00/book   plus shipping and handling.

References

1. J Pharmacol Sci 126, 8-13 (2014) Connection Between Periodontitis and Disease: Possible roles of Microglia and Leptomeningeal
   Cells. Zhov Wu and Hiroshi Nakanishi

2. Hindawi Publishing Corporation Mediators of Inflammation Vol 2013,
   Article ID 407562, 11 pages Leptomeningeal Cells Transduce
Peripheral Macrophages inflammatory Signal to Microglia in Response
to Porphyromonas gingivalis LPs

3. JADA 144 (7) http: // Jada.ada.org July 2013 Gum Disease can raise
your Blood sugar level

4. Pak J Med Sci 2013 Vol 29 No. 1:211-215 doi:
http://dx.doi.org/10.12669/pjms.291.2926 Bidirectional Relationship
between Chronic Kidney Disease & Periodontal Disease Wahid A, et al

5. PNAS September 30, 2003 Vol 150 No 20 11201-11206 Calcification
in Atherosclerosis:Bone biology and chronic inflammation at the arterial
crossroads Doherty, T, et al

6. Clin J Am Soc Nephrol 3: 1598-1605, 20008,
doi:10.2215/CJN.02120508 Media Calcification and Intima Calcification
Are Distinct Entities in Chronic Kidney Disease Amann, K

7. Plos One DOI: 10.1371/Journal.pone. 0114959 Dec 18, 2014
   Serum IgG Antibody Levels to Periodontal Microbiota Are Associated
   With Incident Alzheimer Disease Noble, J, et al

8. The next group of references are all from the J of Periodontol 2013;84 (4 Suppl.): S1-S7,S8-S-19,
The only changes are in the final number following 2013.

The title of the papers are as follows:

Infection and inflammatory mechanisms Van Dyke, TE, et al

Periodontal systemic associations: review of the evidence Linden GJ

The next group of references are continued from the J of Periodontol 2013;84 (4 Suppl.)S20-S23. S24-S29, S30-S50, S51-S60, S61 to S69,

Periodontitis and systemic diseases: a record of discussions of working group 4 of the Joint EFP/AAP Workshop on Periodontitis and Systemic Diseases Linden GJ

Periodontitis and atherosclerotic cardiovascular disease: consensus Report of the Joint EFP/AAP Workshop on Periodontitis and Systemic Diseases Tonetti MS, et al

Periodontal bacterial invasion and infection: contribution to Atherosclerotic pathology Reyes L, et al

Inflammatory mechanisms linking periodontal diseases to cardiovascular diseases Schenkein HA, et al

The next group of references are continued from the J of Periodontol 2013;84 (4 Suppl.) S106-S112, S164-S169, S170-S180,

Diabetes and periodontal diseases: consensus report of the Joint EFP/AAP Workshop on Periodontitis and Systemic Diseases Chapple ILC, Genco R, et al.

Periodontitis and adverse pregnancy outcomes: consensus report of the Joint EFP/AAP Workshop on Periodontitis and Systemic Diseases Sanz M, Kornman K, et al

Adverse pregnancy outcomes (APOs) and periodontal disease: pathogenic Mechanisms Madianos PN, et al

9. J Clin Periodontol 2013: 40 (Suppl. 14) S135-S152
doi:10.1111/jcpe.12080
   Effect of periodontal disease on diabetes: systematic review of
   epidemiologic observational evidence Borgnakke WS, et al.

10.PNAS Sept 30, 2003 Vol. 100 no. 20 11201-11206
   Calcification in atherosclerosis: Bone Biology and chronic
inflammation at the arterial crossroads Doherty TM, et al

11.CLINICAL MICROBIOLOGY REVIEWS, Oct. 2000, p. 547-558 0893-
8512/00/S04.00+0 Vol. 13 No.4
   Systemic Diseases Caused by Oral Infection Xiaojing LI, et al

www.ingramcontent.com/pod-product-compliance
Lightning Source LLC
Chambersburg PA
CBHW070553290526
45790CB00002B/671